DEFEAT COPD

A Comprehensive Guide to Managing and Overcoming Chronic Obstructive Pulmonary Disease

Jessie Williams

CONTENTS

Foreword

Part 1: Living With Chronic Lung Disease

1. When Breathing Becomes Difficult
2. Understanding Lung Disease
3. The Diagnostic Journey

Part 2: The COPD Solution Program

1. Accepting COPD
2. Beginning Oxygen Therapy
3. Breathing Easier
4. Saving Energy
5. Preventing Flare-Ups: Using Medications Effectively
6. Attending Pulmonary Rehabilitation
7. Stopping Smoking
8. Recipes: Eating for Better Breathing
    - Breakfast:

- Whole Grain Bowl
- Greek Granola On-the-Go
- Avocado Breakfast Eggs
- Lunch:
  - Tasty Grilled Cheese
  - Homemade Guacamole
  - Ham and Cream Cheese Roll
- Dinner:
  - Lime Chicken and Rice
  - Quinoa
  - Brown Sugar Salmon
- Desserts/Smoothies:
  - Orange Dream Smoothie
  - Popeye's Favorite Spinach Smoothie
  - Protein Fruit Smoothie
  - Cucumber and Honeydew Smoothie
  - Smoothie on the Beach

9. Practicing Yoga
10. Staying Connected

Common Questions asked by COPD patients and Answers

Vote of Thanks

FOREWORD

Welcome to Defeating COPD, If you or someone close to you has been diagnosed with COPD, this guide is here to offer you the knowledge, strategies, and support needed to handle this challenging condition.

COPD can be an overwhelming diagnosis, but with the right resources and tools, leading a fulfilling and active life is achievable. This ebook blends medical knowledge, practical advice, and personal stories to provide a comprehensive approach to managing COPD. Our goal is to empower you with a deep understanding of the disease, effective treatment plans, and lifestyle adjustments for better health.

Throughout this guide, you'll discover a detailed program designed to help you breathe more easily, save energy, and avoid flare-ups. We'll discuss the advantages of pulmonary rehabilitation, the critical need to quit smoking, and dietary choices that promote better breathing. Moreover, we'll introduce you to exercises like yoga and other methods to boost your overall well-being.

Managing COPD requires a holistic approach, and we hope this guide becomes a valuable resource in your battle against this disease. Remember, you are not alone—support, information, and assistance are available at every step.

We encourage you to take charge of your health and join us in defeating COPD. Together, we can significantly improve your quality of life.

Warm regards,
Jessie Wiiliams

PART 1
Living With Chronic Lung Disease

CHAPTER 1: WHEN BREATHING BECOMES DIFFICULT

Chronic Obstructive Pulmonary Disease (COPD) is a multifaceted, progressive condition impacting millions globally. It includes respiratory illnesses such as chronic bronchitis and emphysema, which gradually deteriorate lung function. This chapter explores the experience of living with chronic lung disease, emphasizing the personal and physical difficulties encountered when breathing becomes challenging.

Understanding COPD

COPD is marked by ongoing respiratory symptoms and airflow restriction due to abnormalities in the airways and/or alveoli. These issues generally arise from prolonged exposure to harmful particles or gases. The primary cause is cigarette smoking, though other risks include long-term exposure to air pollution, chemical fumes, and dust. Genetic factors, like alpha-1 antitrypsin deficiency, also contribute to some cases.

Symptoms of COPD often begin subtly and progressively worsen. They include a persistent cough, frequent respiratory infections, shortness of breath (particularly during physical activity), wheezing, and chest tightness. As the disease advances, these symptoms can become more severe and significantly diminish the quality of life.

The Daily Reality of Living with COPD

Imagine starting each day with a feeling of heaviness in your chest. Routine activities, such as getting out of bed, brushing your teeth, or preparing breakfast, become monumental tasks. For those with COPD, this is a constant reality. The struggle for air creates a persistent sense of anxiety and fear, aware that the next exacerbation could result in hospitalization or worse.

Morning Routine

For many, managing their condition begins with a morning routine. This typically involves taking prescribed medications, like bronchodilators and inhaled steroids, to open the airways and reduce inflammation. Morning exercises, such as controlled breathing techniques and gentle stretches, help loosen mucus and enhance lung function.

Despite these measures, there are good and bad days. On bad days, even simple tasks can be exhausting. The unpredictability of symptoms adds to the psychological burden, making it hard to plan daily activities or social events.

Managing Symptoms Throughout the Day

Living with COPD requires constant vigilance and adaptation. Symptoms can be triggered or worsened by various factors, including weather changes, pollutant exposure, infections, and physical exertion. Therefore, monitoring the environment and making necessary adjustments is crucial.

Physical Challenges

1. Breathlessness: One of the most distressing symptoms of COPD is dyspnea, or breathlessness. This can

occur even at rest in advanced stages, making activities like walking, climbing stairs, or even talking difficult. Patients often have to adopt a slower pace and take frequent breaks.

2. Fatigue: Chronic fatigue is another common issue. The extra effort required to breathe can leave patients feeling exhausted. This can lead to a vicious cycle where reduced activity leads to muscle deconditioning, further exacerbating breathlessness and fatigue.

3. Frequent Infections: People with COPD are more susceptible to respiratory infections, which can cause severe exacerbations. These infections often require antibiotics or antiviral

medications and can result in hospitalization.

Psychological Challenges

1. Anxiety and Depression: The chronic nature of COPD, combined with the physical limitations and uncertainty of the disease, can lead to significant anxiety and depression. Patients may feel isolated, frustrated, and fearful of the future.

2. Social Isolation: The physical limitations and the need to avoid triggers can lead to social withdrawal. Patients might avoid activities they once enjoyed, leading to feelings of loneliness and social isolation.

3. Coping Mechanisms: Developing effective coping mechanisms is crucial for managing the psychological impact of COPD. Support groups, counseling, and cognitive-behavioral therapy (CBT) can be beneficial.

The Importance of a Support System

Living with COPD is not something that should be done alone. The importance of a strong support system cannot be overstated. Family members, friends, and healthcare providers play crucial roles in providing physical assistance, emotional support, and medical care.

Family and Friends

The role of family and friends is pivotal. They can assist with daily tasks, provide transportation to medical appointments, and offer emotional support. Understanding the nature of COPD and the challenges it brings can help them be more empathetic and supportive.

Healthcare Team

A comprehensive healthcare team typically includes a primary care physician, pulmonologist, respiratory therapist, physical therapist, and possibly a mental health professional. Regular check-ups, pulmonary function tests, and adherence to treatment plans are essential for managing the disease.

Support Groups

Joining a support group can provide a sense of community and understanding. Sharing experiences with others who are facing similar challenges can be comforting and empowering. Support groups can also offer practical advice and coping strategies.

Adapting to a New Lifestyle

Adapting to life with COPD requires significant lifestyle changes. These changes are aimed at managing symptoms, preventing exacerbations, and maintaining as much independence and quality of life as possible.

Smoking Cessation

If you are a smoker, quitting is the most critical step you can take. Smoking cessation can slow the progression of COPD and improve your symptoms. There are various resources available, including counseling, medications, and support groups, to help you quit.

Healthy Diet and Exercise

Eating a balanced diet and maintaining a healthy weight are important. A diet rich in fruits, vegetables, lean proteins, and whole grains can provide the necessary nutrients to support your body. Avoiding foods that can cause bloating or discomfort is also essential, as a full stomach can make breathing more difficult.

Exercise, particularly pulmonary rehabilitation programs, can improve your overall fitness and lung function. These programs often include aerobic exercises, strength training, and breathing exercises designed specifically for people with COPD.

Medication Adherence

Taking medications as prescribed is crucial. This includes not only bronchodilators and steroids but also vaccinations against influenza and pneumonia, which can prevent serious infections.

Avoiding Triggers

Identifying and avoiding triggers is a key part of managing COPD. This might include staying indoors on days with high air pollution or pollen counts, avoiding exposure to chemical fumes or smoke, and taking precautions to avoid infections.

The Road Ahead

While living with COPD presents many challenges, it is possible to manage the disease and maintain a good quality of life. Education, proactive management, and a strong support system are essential. Advances in medical treatment and a better understanding of the disease offer hope for improved outcomes.

In the chapters that follow, we will explore these strategies in more detail, providing practical advice and guidance on managing COPD. From understanding the latest treatments to learning effective breathing techniques and making lifestyle adjustments, this book aims to equip you with the knowledge and tools you need to live well with COPD.

When breathing becomes difficult, it is natural to feel overwhelmed and anxious. But with the right approach and support, you can take control of your health and lead a fulfilling life despite the challenges of COPD. The journey may be challenging, but it is

not one you have to face alone.
Together, we can defeat COPD.

CHAPTER 2: UNDERSTANDING LUNG DISEASE

Chronic Obstructive Pulmonary Disease (COPD) refers to a collection of progressive lung conditions, including chronic bronchitis and emphysema. To effectively manage and overcome COPD, it is crucial to understand the nature of these lung diseases, their causes, symptoms, and how they impact the respiratory system. This chapter offers a detailed overview of lung diseases, focusing on COPD, to help you comprehend the challenges you face and the importance of proactive management.

The Structure and Function of the Lungs

The lungs, a pair of spongy, air-filled organs located in the chest, facilitate the exchange of oxygen and carbon dioxide between the air and the blood. The breathing process involves several key components:

1. Airways: Comprising the trachea (windpipe) and a network of branching tubes called bronchi and bronchioles, these structures transport air in and out of the lungs.
2. Alveoli: Tiny air sacs at the end of the bronchioles where gas exchange takes place. Oxygen moves through the alveolar walls into the blood vessels,

while carbon dioxide passes from the blood into the alveoli to be exhaled.
3. Diaphragm: A dome-shaped muscle at the lung base that plays a crucial role in breathing. When the diaphragm contracts, it creates a vacuum that draws air into the lungs. When it relaxes, air is expelled.

In healthy lungs, this process is efficient, ensuring the body receives the necessary oxygen. However, in individuals with lung disease, this process is impaired, leading to various symptoms and complications.

What is COPD?

COPD is a chronic inflammatory lung disease that obstructs airflow from the lungs. It is progressive, meaning it worsens over time. The two primary forms of COPD are:

1. Chronic Bronchitis: Involves inflammation of the bronchial tube lining, leading to excessive mucus production, which can obstruct the airways and complicate breathing. Chronic bronchitis is diagnosed when a person has a productive cough (producing mucus) lasting for at least three months in two consecutive years.

2. Emphysema: Involves damage to the alveoli, the tiny air sacs in the lungs.

The destruction of the walls between alveoli creates larger but fewer air sacs, reducing the surface area for gas exchange. This leads to shortness of breath and decreased oxygen supply to the bloodstream.

Most individuals with COPD have a combination of both chronic bronchitis and emphysema.

Causes and Risk Factors

The main cause of COPD is long-term exposure to irritating gases or particulate matter, primarily from cigarette smoke. Other factors contributing to COPD include:

1. Smoking: The most significant risk factor, with about 85-90% of COPD cases attributed to smoking.
2. Secondhand Smoke: Prolonged exposure to secondhand smoke also increases the risk of COPD.
3. Occupational Exposure: Exposure to dust, chemicals, and fumes in the workplace can contribute to COPD.
4. Air Pollution: Long-term exposure to air pollution can increase the risk of developing COPD.
5. Genetics: A rare genetic disorder called alpha-1 antitrypsin deficiency can cause COPD, affecting the body's ability to produce a protein that protects the lungs.
6. Respiratory Infections: Severe respiratory infections in childhood can increase the risk of COPD later in life.

Symptoms of COPD

COPD symptoms develop gradually and may not be noticeable until significant lung damage has occurred. Key symptoms include:

1. Chronic Cough: Often the first symptom, it may produce mucus (sputum) that can be clear, white, yellow, or greenish.
2. Shortness of Breath: Especially during physical activities, which can progress to breathlessness even at rest as the disease advances.
3. Wheezing: A whistling or squeaky sound when breathing.
4. Chest Tightness: A feeling of constriction or pressure in the chest.

5. Frequent Respiratory Infections: Increased susceptibility to colds, flu, and other respiratory infections.

6. Fatigue: Persistent tiredness due to the extra effort required to breathe.

7. Blueness of the Lips or Fingernail Beds: Also known as cyanosis, indicating low oxygen levels in the blood.

Diagnosis of COPD

Diagnosing COPD involves a combination of medical history, physical examination, and diagnostic tests. Common diagnostic methods include:

1. Spirometry: The most common test for diagnosing COPD. It measures the

amount of air a person can inhale and exhale and how quickly they can exhale, helping to determine the severity of the disease.

2. Chest X-ray: Can reveal emphysema and rule out other lung problems or heart failure.

3. CT Scan: Provides detailed images of the lungs and can help detect emphysema and determine if surgery is needed.

4. Arterial Blood Gas Analysis: Measures the oxygen and carbon dioxide levels in the blood, indicating lung function.

5. Alpha-1 Antitrypsin Deficiency Screening: A blood test to determine if a genetic deficiency is contributing to COPD.

The Impact of COPD on Daily Life

Living with COPD affects all aspects of daily life, from physical capabilities to emotional well-being. As the disease progresses, symptoms worsen, making everyday activities increasingly difficult.

Physical Impact

1. Reduced Physical Activity: Breathlessness and fatigue can limit physical activity, leading to muscle weakness and deconditioning, which in turn can worsen breathlessness and create a cycle of declining physical health.

2. Frequent Exacerbations: Symptom flare-ups, known as exacerbations, can be triggered by infections, pollutants, or other irritants. These exacerbations can be severe, requiring hospitalization and causing further lung damage.

3. Need for Supplemental Oxygen: In advanced stages, some people may require supplemental oxygen to maintain adequate oxygen levels in the blood.

Psychological and Emotional Impact

1. Anxiety and Depression: The chronic nature and physical limitations of COPD can lead to significant anxiety and depression. Fear of exacerbations, social isolation, and the stress of managing a chronic illness contribute to mental health challenges.

2. Social Isolation: Physical limitations and the need to avoid environmental triggers can lead to social withdrawal and feelings of loneliness.

3. Coping Mechanisms: Effective coping strategies, including support groups, counseling, and cognitive-behavioral therapy (CBT), are crucial for managing the psychological impact of COPD.

The Importance of Early Detection and Management

Early detection and proactive management of COPD are vital to slowing disease progression, reducing symptoms, and improving quality of life. Key management strategies include:

Smoking Cessation

For smokers, quitting is the most important step. Smoking cessation can slow the progression of COPD and improve symptoms. Resources such as counseling, medications, and support groups can assist in quitting.

Medications

Medications are essential for managing COPD symptoms and preventing exacerbations. These may include:

1. Bronchodilators: Help relax the muscles around the airways, making breathing easier.
2. Inhaled Corticosteroids: Reduce inflammation in the airways.
3. Combination Inhalers: Combine bronchodilators and corticosteroids.
4. Antibiotics: Used to treat respiratory infections that can exacerbate COPD symptoms.
5. Vaccinations: Annual flu vaccines and pneumococcal vaccines to prevent respiratory infections.

Pulmonary Rehabilitation

Pulmonary rehabilitation programs combine exercise training, education, and support to help manage COPD symptoms and improve overall health. These programs focus on:

1. Exercise Training: Tailored exercises to improve cardiovascular fitness and muscle strength.
2. Breathing Exercises: Techniques to improve breathing efficiency and reduce breathlessness.
3. Nutritional Counseling: Guidance on maintaining a healthy diet to support overall health and energy levels.
4. Education: Information on managing symptoms, using medications correctly, and recognizing signs of exacerbations.

Lifestyle Modifications

Making lifestyle changes can significantly impact COPD management and quality of life. These include:

1. Healthy Diet: Eating a balanced diet rich in fruits, vegetables, lean proteins, and whole grains supports overall health and energy levels.
2. Regular Exercise: Engaging in regular physical activity, tailored to individual capabilities, helps maintain muscle strength and cardiovascular fitness.
3. Avoiding Triggers: Identifying and avoiding environmental triggers, such as air pollution, smoke, and chemical fumes, helps reduce the risk of exacerbations.

Psychological Support

Addressing the psychological impact of COPD is crucial for overall well-being. This can include:

1. Support Groups: Joining support groups provides a sense of community and understanding, helping to alleviate feelings of isolation.
2. Counseling: Professional counseling can help manage anxiety, depression, and stress related to COPD.
3. Cognitive-Behavioral Therapy (CBT): CBT techniques can help develop effective coping strategies and improve mental health.

Conclusion

Understanding lung disease, particularly COPD, is the first step toward effective management and improved quality of life. By recognizing the symptoms, causes, and impact of COPD, you can take proactive measures to manage the disease and maintain your health.

CHAPTER 3: THE DIAGNOSTIC JOURNEY

Among chronic illnesses, the diagnosis of Chronic Obstructive Pulmonary Disease (COPD) can be particularly intimidating. The process to identify and confirm this condition involves a detailed diagnostic journey with numerous tests, assessments, and consultations. Knowing what this journey entails can help you navigate it more effectively and adopt a proactive stance towards managing your health. This chapter delves into the diagnostic process for COPD, from recognizing initial symptoms to receiving a confirmed diagnosis, emphasizing the importance of each step and outlining what you can expect throughout.

Recognizing Symptoms and Seeking Help

The diagnostic process usually starts when symptoms are first noticed. COPD symptoms often develop gradually and can be confused with other conditions or attributed to aging. Early symptoms include a persistent cough, breathlessness during physical activity, wheezing, chest tightness, and increased mucus production. As these symptoms worsen, they can significantly disrupt daily life, prompting individuals to seek medical advice.

Recognizing these symptoms early and consulting a healthcare professional promptly is crucial. Many people delay seeking help until the disease has progressed, complicating management. If you experience these symptoms, particularly if you have risk factors such as a smoking history or exposure to lung irritants, it's essential to consult a healthcare provider without delay.

Initial Medical Consultation

The first step in diagnosing COPD is an initial consultation with a healthcare provider, often your primary care physician. During this visit, your doctor will take a detailed medical history, asking about your symptoms, their duration and severity, and any risk factors. They will also conduct a physical examination, listening to your lungs with a stethoscope for abnormal sounds like wheezing or crackling.

Your doctor might ask about your smoking history, occupational exposures, family history of respiratory diseases, and any past respiratory infections. Providing accurate and detailed information during this consultation is crucial, as it helps your doctor assess the likelihood of COPD and decide on the next steps in the diagnostic process.

Diagnostic Tests

If COPD is suspected based on your symptoms and medical history, your healthcare provider will recommend several diagnostic tests to confirm the diagnosis and determine the disease's severity. These tests are vital for gaining a comprehensive understanding of your lung function and overall health.

Spirometry

Spirometry is the most common and essential test for diagnosing COPD. It measures the volume of air you can inhale and exhale, and how quickly you can exhale. During this test, you will take a deep breath and blow into a mouthpiece connected to a spirometer. This device records the air volume and flow, providing critical information about your lung function.

Key measurements from spirometry include:

1. Forced Vital Capacity (FVC): The total amount of air you can exhale after taking a deep breath.
2. Forced Expiratory Volume in one second (FEV1): The amount of air you can forcefully exhale in the first second.

The ratio of FEV1 to FVC is used to diagnose COPD. A lower ratio indicates airflow obstruction, a key feature of COPD. Spirometry is not only used for diagnosis but also for monitoring disease progression and treatment effectiveness over time.

Chest X-ray

A chest X-ray is a standard imaging test used to visualize the lungs and identify any abnormalities. While a chest X-ray cannot definitively diagnose COPD, it can help rule out other conditions like pneumonia, lung cancer, or heart failure that might cause similar symptoms. In individuals with COPD, a chest X-ray may show signs of emphysema, such as enlarged lungs and a flattened diaphragm, or chronic bronchitis, such as thickened bronchial walls.

CT Scan

A computed tomography (CT) scan offers more detailed images of the lungs compared to a chest X-ray. It can detect emphysema, assess lung damage extent, and identify other lung conditions not visible on a standard X-ray. A CT scan is particularly useful for planning treatments like lung volume reduction surgery or assessing the need for more invasive diagnostic procedures.

Arterial Blood Gas Analysis

Arterial blood gas (ABG) analysis measures oxygen and carbon dioxide levels in your blood, providing critical information about lung function. This test involves drawing a small blood sample from an artery, usually in the wrist. ABG analysis is particularly useful for assessing COPD severity and determining if supplemental oxygen is needed.

Pulse Oximetry

Pulse oximetry is a non-invasive test that measures blood oxygen saturation levels. A small sensor is placed on your fingertip or earlobe, using light to estimate the oxygen percentage in your blood. While not as detailed as ABG analysis, pulse oximetry is a quick and easy way to assess your oxygen levels and is often used alongside other tests.

Alpha-1 Antitrypsin Deficiency Screening

Alpha-1 antitrypsin deficiency is a rare genetic disorder that can cause COPD. This condition affects the body's ability to produce alpha-1 antitrypsin, a protein that protects the lungs from damage. If diagnosed with COPD at a young age or if there is a family history of the disease, your doctor may recommend a blood test to screen for this deficiency. Identifying alpha-1 antitrypsin deficiency is important because it can affect COPD management and treatment.

Specialist Consultation

In some cases, your primary care physician may refer you to a pulmonologist, a specialist in lung diseases, for further evaluation and management. A pulmonologist can provide more specialized care, including advanced diagnostic tests and treatments. They may also manage complex COPD cases or when the disease does not respond well to standard treatments.

Interpreting the Results and Confirming the Diagnosis

Once all diagnostic tests are completed, your healthcare provider will review the results with you. A confirmed COPD diagnosis is based on a combination of your medical history, physical examination, and test results, particularly spirometry. COPD severity is often classified into stages based on the GOLD (Global Initiative for Chronic Obstructive Lung Disease) criteria, which consider FEV1 values and symptom severity. These stages range from mild (GOLD 1) to very severe (GOLD 4).

The GOLD Staging System

1. GOLD 1 (Mild): FEV1 ≥ 80% predicted. Symptoms are usually mild, including a chronic cough and increased mucus production.
2. GOLD 2 (Moderate): FEV1 50-79% predicted. Symptoms become more noticeable, with increased shortness of breath during physical activities.
3. GOLD 3 (Severe): FEV1 30-49% predicted. Symptoms are more severe, significantly limiting physical activity and causing frequent exacerbations.
4. GOLD 4 (Very Severe): FEV1 < 30% predicted. Symptoms are severe and persistent, with a high risk of life-

threatening exacerbations and respiratory failure.

Understanding your COPD stage is crucial for creating an effective management plan tailored to your specific needs.

The Emotional Impact of Diagnosis

Receiving a COPD diagnosis can be overwhelming and emotionally taxing. It's common to experience a range of emotions, including fear, anxiety, sadness, and frustration. Acknowledging and addressing these feelings is an important part of the diagnostic journey. Seeking support from family, friends, support groups, or a mental health professional can help you cope with the emotional impact of the diagnosis and adjust to life changes.

Conclusion

The diagnostic journey for COPD is a critical first step in understanding and managing the disease. From recognizing symptoms and seeking medical help to undergoing diagnostic tests and receiving a confirmed diagnosis, each step is essential in developing an effective management plan. By understanding the diagnostic process and adopting a proactive approach to your health, you can take control of your COPD and work towards a better quality of life.

Part 2
The COPD Solution Program

CHAPTER 1: ACCEPTING COPD

Acceptance is essential for managing any chronic illness, and Chronic Obstructive Pulmonary Disease (COPD) is no exception. Embracing your condition with a proactive mindset can greatly impact your ability to handle the disease and enhance your quality of life. This chapter explores the importance of accepting COPD, the psychological aspects of chronic illness, and practical strategies to maintain a positive outlook. Accepting COPD is not about surrendering; rather, it involves recognizing your condition, understanding its implications, and taking actionable steps to live a meaningful life despite the challenges.

Understanding COPD

COPD is a progressive lung disease that makes breathing difficult. It includes conditions such as emphysema and chronic bronchitis, characterized by persistent airflow obstruction. Common symptoms are chronic cough, shortness of breath, wheezing, and frequent respiratory infections. Long-term exposure to lung irritants, primarily cigarette smoke, is the main cause of COPD. Other causes include air pollution, chemical fumes, and dust.

Understanding COPD is the first step toward acceptance. Educate yourself about the disease, its symptoms, progression, and treatment options. Knowledge empowers you and can demystify the condition, making it less intimidating. By learning about COPD, you can better understand what to expect and how to manage your symptoms effectively.

The Psychological Impact of COPD

A COPD diagnosis can be overwhelming, and it's normal to experience a range of emotions such as fear, anger, sadness, and frustration. The chronic nature of the disease and its impact on daily life can lead to feelings of loss and anxiety. Addressing these emotional responses is vital for acceptance and effective disease management.

Common Emotional Reactions

- Denial: Initially, you might find it hard to accept your COPD diagnosis, especially if you were previously healthy. Denial can serve as a protective mechanism, but prolonged denial can hinder effective disease management.
- Anger: You might feel angry about your diagnosis, particularly if you have lived a healthy lifestyle or avoided smoking. Anger can be directed at yourself, others, or the situation.

- Depression: Chronic illnesses like COPD can lead to depression, characterized by feelings of hopelessness, loss of interest in activities, and persistent sadness. Depression can negatively impact your motivation to manage the disease and overall quality of life.
- Anxiety: The uncertainty of living with a chronic condition can cause anxiety, with concerns about symptom management, disease progression, and its impact on daily life being overwhelming.

Coping with Emotions

Acknowledging and addressing these emotions is crucial for progress. Here are strategies to cope with the psychological impact of COPD:

- Seek Support: Talking to family, friends, or support groups can provide emotional relief and practical advice. Sharing experiences with those who understand can help reduce feelings of isolation.
- Professional Help: Consider seeking help from a mental health professional. Therapists or counselors can offer strategies to manage your emotions and develop coping mechanisms.
-Mindfulness and Relaxation: Practices such as mindfulness meditation, deep breathing exercises, and progressive muscle relaxation can help reduce stress and anxiety, improving your ability to manage COPD symptoms.

- Stay Active: Physical activity can boost your mood and overall well-being. Engage in activities you enjoy and are within your physical capabilities.

Embracing a Positive Mindset

Accepting COPD involves adopting a positive and proactive mindset. While it's essential to acknowledge the challenges, focusing on what you can control can make a significant difference in your quality of life. Here are some ways to cultivate a positive outlook:

Set Realistic Goals

Setting achievable goals provides a sense of purpose and direction. Start with small, manageable objectives related to your health and daily activities. As you achieve these goals, you can gradually set more challenging ones. Celebrating your progress, no matter how small, can boost your confidence and motivation.

Focus on What You Can Control

While you cannot change your COPD diagnosis, you can control how you manage the disease. Focus on actions that can improve your symptoms and overall well-being, such as adhering to your treatment plan, maintaining a healthy lifestyle, and staying active. By taking control of your health, you can enhance your quality of life.

Educate Yourself

Knowledge is empowering. Educate yourself about COPD, treatment options, and strategies to manage symptoms. Stay informed about new research and advancements in COPD care. The more you know, the better equipped you will be to make informed decisions about your health.

Build a Support Network

Surround yourself with supportive and understanding individuals, including family, friends, healthcare providers, and support groups. A strong support network can provide emotional support, practical advice, and encouragement when you need it most.

Practice Self-Compassion

Be kind to yourself. Living with COPD can be challenging, and it's important to acknowledge your efforts and progress. Avoid self-criticism and recognize that managing a chronic illness is a journey with ups and downs. Practice self-compassion and give yourself credit for your resilience and determination.

Developing a Plan

Accepting COPD also means developing a comprehensive plan to manage the disease. This includes working closely with your healthcare team to create a personalized treatment plan, setting realistic goals, and establishing a routine that supports your health.

Create a Treatment Plan

Work with your healthcare providers to develop a treatment plan tailored to your specific needs. This plan should include medications, pulmonary rehabilitation, lifestyle changes, and regular check-ups. Adhering to your treatment plan is crucial for managing symptoms and preventing exacerbations.

Set Up a Routine

Establish a daily routine that incorporates activities to support your health. This includes taking medications as prescribed, engaging in physical activity, following a healthy diet, and practicing relaxation techniques. A consistent routine can help you manage COPD more effectively and improve your overall well-being.

Monitor Your Symptoms

Regularly monitor your symptoms and keep track of any changes. This can help you and your healthcare team identify patterns and make necessary adjustments to your treatment plan. Use a symptom diary or mobile app to log your symptoms, medications, and any triggers.

Stay Informed

Stay up-to-date with the latest information and advancements in COPD care. Attend educational workshops, read reputable sources, and participate in support groups. Staying informed empowers you to make informed decisions about your health and treatment options.

Conclusion

Accepting COPD is a critical step in managing the disease and improving your quality of life. It involves acknowledging the reality of your condition, understanding its impact, and adopting a proactive and positive mindset. By addressing the psychological aspects of COPD, embracing a positive outlook, and developing a comprehensive management plan, you can take control of your health and live a fulfilling life despite the challenges of COPD. Remember, acceptance is not about giving up; it's about empowering yourself to manage the disease and thrive.

CHAPTER 2: BEGINNING OXYGEN THERAPY

Oxygen therapy plays a vital role in the management of Chronic Obstructive Pulmonary Disease (COPD) for many individuals. This chapter explores the importance of oxygen therapy, its benefits, considerations, and practical advice for integrating it into daily life. Understanding how oxygen therapy functions, when it's necessary, and how to effectively utilize it can significantly improve COPD management and enhance overall well-being.

Understanding Oxygen Therapy

Oxygen therapy involves administering supplemental oxygen to increase oxygen levels in the bloodstream. In COPD, the lungs often struggle to absorb sufficient oxygen from the air, resulting in low blood oxygen levels (hypoxemia). Oxygen therapy helps correct this imbalance, ensuring organs and tissues receive adequate oxygen supply.

Indications for Oxygen Therapy

Oxygen therapy is typically prescribed for COPD patients with low blood oxygen levels, usually determined through arterial blood gas (ABG) analysis. Key indications include:

- Resting Hypoxemia: Low oxygen levels while at rest, typically indicated by an arterial oxygen saturation (SaO2) of 88% or lower.
- Exercise-Induced Hypoxemia: Low oxygen levels during physical activity, which can severely limit daily activities.

- Chronic Respiratory Failure: Severe COPD leading to chronically low oxygen levels despite other treatments.

Your healthcare provider will assess your oxygen levels and determine the need for oxygen therapy based on your symptoms, test results, and overall health status.

Types of Oxygen Delivery Systems

Several oxygen delivery systems are available to effectively administer supplemental oxygen:

- Oxygen Concentrators: Electrically powered devices that extract oxygen from the air and deliver it via a nasal cannula or mask. Oxygen concentrators are suitable for continuous use at home.

- Portable Oxygen Tanks: Store compressed oxygen gas delivered through portable cylinders or tanks. These are convenient for COPD patients needing oxygen on the go, especially where electrical access may be limited.

- Liquid Oxygen Systems: Store oxygen in liquid form, converting it to gas for inhalation. These systems are portable and refillable as needed.

- Oxygen Conservers: Devices that regulate oxygen flow based on breathing patterns, conserving oxygen and extending the use of portable tanks or liquid oxygen.

Benefits of Oxygen Therapy

Oxygen therapy provides numerous advantages for individuals with COPD:

- Improved Oxygenation: Correcting low blood oxygen levels enhances oxygen delivery to organs and tissues, reducing symptoms such as breathlessness and fatigue.

- Enhanced Quality of Life: Adequate oxygenation supports physical activities, allowing for greater independence and participation in social and recreational pursuits.

- Reduced Complications: Supplemental oxygen helps prevent complications associated with chronic hypoxemia, such as pulmonary hypertension and heart failure.

- Better Sleep Quality: Oxygen therapy alleviates nighttime hypoxemia, improving sleep patterns and reducing symptoms like morning headaches and daytime tiredness.

Beginning Oxygen Therapy

Initiating oxygen therapy is a significant milestone in COPD management. Here are practical considerations and steps to ensure a smooth transition to oxygen therapy:

Consultation with Your Healthcare Provider

Upon recommendation for oxygen therapy, discuss the following with your healthcare provider:

- Prescription Details: Understand the prescribed oxygen flow rate (liters per minute) and therapy duration (continuous or as needed).

- Oxygen Delivery System: Select the most suitable system based on your lifestyle and needs (e.g., home-use concentrator, portable tanks for mobility).

- Safety Guidelines: Familiarize yourself with safety precautions, including fire safety (oxygen supports combustion) and proper storage practices.

- Monitoring: Establish a follow-up schedule to monitor oxygen levels, adjust settings if necessary, and address any questions or concerns.

Getting Started with Oxygen Equipment

Once prescribed, become proficient with your oxygen equipment:

- Oxygen Concentrator: Learn to set up, operate, and maintain the concentrator according to manufacturer guidelines.

- Portable Tanks: Understand safe handling, transportation, and refilling procedures for portable oxygen tanks.

- Oxygen Delivery Devices: Practice using nasal cannulas, masks, or other devices as instructed to ensure proper oxygen delivery and comfort.

Integrating Oxygen Therapy into Daily Life

Incorporating oxygen therapy into your routine requires planning and adjustment:

- Mobility: Plan activities around oxygen needs, ensuring access to oxygen wherever you go. Utilize portable tanks or liquid oxygen systems for outings or travel.

- Safety:!Adhere to safety guidelines, including avoiding smoking or open flames near oxygen equipment and ensuring adequate ventilation in confined spaces.

- Support System: Educate family, caregivers, or close contacts about oxygen therapy requirements, emergency protocols, and signs of potential complications.

Monitoring and Adjustment

Regularly monitor symptoms and oxygen saturation levels to assess therapy effectiveness:

- Symptom Management: Maintain a symptom journal to track changes in breathlessness, fatigue, and other COPD symptoms. Report any worsening symptoms promptly to your healthcare provider.

- Oxygen Saturation: Use a pulse oximeter regularly, especially during physical activity or altitude changes, to monitor oxygen levels.

- Follow-up Care: Attend scheduled appointments to review progress, adjust oxygen settings if necessary, and discuss any concerns or questions with your healthcare provider.

Conclusion

Beginning oxygen therapy is a crucial step in effectively managing COPD and enhancing quality of life. By understanding the role of oxygen therapy, selecting appropriate delivery systems, and integrating therapy into daily routines, individuals with COPD can better manage symptoms, participate more fully in daily activities, and reduce risks associated with chronic hypoxemia. Close collaboration with healthcare providers, adherence to safety guidelines, and staying informed about oxygen therapy protocols are essential for maximizing therapy benefits and achieving improved COPD management outcomes. Remember, oxygen therapy is a supportive tool that empowers individuals to live fulfilling lives despite the challenges of COPD.

CHAPTER 3: BREATHING EASIER

Improving respiratory function and reducing breathlessness are primary objectives for individuals managing Chronic Obstructive Pulmonary Disease (COPD). This chapter explores a variety of strategies, techniques, and lifestyle adjustments aimed at achieving these goals and enhancing overall quality of life. By integrating these practices with The COPD Solution Program, individuals can effectively manage their symptoms and experience greater comfort in their daily lives.

Understanding COPD Symptoms

COPD manifests through several symptoms that significantly impact respiratory function and daily activities:

- Chronic Cough: Persistent coughing accompanied by mucus production is a common symptom.
- Shortness of Breath (Dyspnea): Breathlessness, especially during physical exertion or daily tasks, is a hallmark indicator of COPD.
- Wheezing: High-pitched whistling sounds during breathing due to narrowed airways.

- Chest Tightness: Discomfort or pressure in the chest area, often exacerbated during exacerbations.
- Fatigue: Feeling tired or lacking energy, often associated with reduced oxygen levels.

Understanding and effectively managing these symptoms are crucial for improving respiratory function and overall well-being.

Strategies for Breathing Easier

1. Quitting Smoking

Smoking cessation stands as the most effective intervention for slowing COPD progression and improving lung function. Emphasized in The COPD Solution Program, quitting smoking reduces airway inflammation, decreases mucus production, and slows lung function decline. Support from healthcare providers, smoking cessation programs, and behavioral counseling significantly enhances success rates in quitting smoking.

2. Adhering to Medication

Strict adherence to prescribed medications is critical for managing COPD symptoms and preventing exacerbations. The COPD Solution Program features a comprehensive medication plan tailored to individual needs, including bronchodilators, corticosteroids, antibiotics for exacerbations, and mucolytic agents to reduce mucus production. Following medication schedules as prescribed ensures optimal symptom control and improves respiratory function.

3. Engaging in Pulmonary Rehabilitation

Pulmonary rehabilitation is a structured program integral to managing COPD symptoms, enhancing exercise tolerance, and improving overall quality of life. Typically encompassing exercise training, education on COPD management, breathing techniques, and nutritional counseling, pulmonary rehabilitation in The COPD Solution Program helps individuals strengthen respiratory muscles, enhance lung capacity, and manage breathlessness during daily activities effectively.

4. Mastering Breathing Techniques

Learning and practicing effective breathing techniques significantly aid in managing breathlessness and enhancing oxygenation:

- Pursed Lip Breathing: Inhaling slowly through the nose and exhaling through pursed lips as if blowing out a candle helps keep airways open longer and reduces breathing effort.

- Diaphragmatic Breathing: Also known as belly or abdominal breathing, this technique involves deep inhalation through the nose, allowing the abdomen to rise, followed by slow exhalation through pursed lips. Diaphragmatic breathing strengthens the diaphragm muscle and improves overall lung function.

5. Embracing Physical Activity

Regular physical activity plays a pivotal role in improving cardiovascular health, increasing muscle strength, and boosting endurance for individuals with COPD. The COPD Solution Program incorporates tailored exercise regimens featuring aerobic exercises (such as walking and cycling) and strength training to enhance respiratory muscle strength. Supervised physical activity helps manage breathlessness and enhances overall fitness levels.

6. Optimizing Nutrition

Maintaining a balanced diet rich in nutrients supports overall health and enhances respiratory function. The COPD Solution Program advises on:

- Healthy Fats: Incorporating omega-3 fatty acids from sources like fish, nuts, and seeds to reduce airway inflammation.

- Lean Proteins: Protein-rich foods such as lean meats, poultry, beans, and legumes support muscle strength and repair.

- Fruits and Vegetables: Colorful produce provides antioxidants that reduce oxidative stress and inflammation in the lungs.

7. Environmental Adaptations

Reducing exposure to environmental irritants and pollutants aids in managing COPD symptoms and preventing exacerbations:

- Indoor Air Quality: Ensuring adequate ventilation, using air purifiers as needed, and avoiding smoke, strong odors, and chemical fumes.

- Outdoor Precautions: Limiting outdoor activities during high pollution or allergen days. Using a mask or scarf over the nose and mouth in cold weather helps warm and humidify inhaled air.

8. Emotional and Psychological Support

Coping with COPD involves managing emotional and psychological challenges. The COPD Solution Program emphasizes mental health support and coping strategies:

- Support Networks: Participating in COPD support groups or online communities provides peer support, shared experiences, and practical advice for managing the emotional impact of COPD.

- Stress Management: Techniques such as meditation, deep breathing exercises, and mindfulness reduce stress levels and enhance coping mechanisms.

- Counseling Services: Professional counseling or therapy helps individuals address anxiety, depression, or adjustment issues associated with chronic illness.

Conclusion

Achieving easier breathing is attainable for individuals with COPD through proactive management strategies outlined in The COPD Solution Program. By focusing on smoking cessation, medication adherence, pulmonary rehabilitation, breathing techniques, physical activity, nutrition, environmental modifications, and emotional support, individuals can effectively manage symptoms, enhance respiratory function, and improve quality of life. The comprehensive framework provided empowers individuals to take control of their health and well-being despite the challenges posed by COPD. Through dedication, support, and informed decision-making, individuals with COPD can achieve greater comfort, independence, and a fulfilling life.

CHAPTER 4: ACCEPTING AND SAVING ENERGY

Recognizing the necessity of conserving energy is a critical component of effectively managing Chronic Obstructive Pulmonary Disease (COPD). This chapter delves into the importance of energy conservation, practical strategies to reduce exertion, and tips for seamlessly integrating these practices into daily life. By adopting energy-saving techniques in conjunction with The COPD Solution Program, individuals can enhance their daily activities, better manage symptoms, and ultimately improve their overall quality of life.

Understanding Energy Conservation in COPD

Energy conservation entails managing and preserving physical and mental energy to minimize fatigue and optimize daily functioning. For individuals grappling with COPD, conserving energy is paramount due to the heightened effort required for breathing and physical tasks. Symptoms like breathlessness and fatigue can exacerbate with exertion, making it challenging to accomplish tasks without experiencing excessive tiredness.

Impact of COPD on Energy Levels

COPD impacts energy levels in several ways:

- Increased Energy Expenditure: Breathing becomes more arduous due to narrowed airways and reduced lung function, necessitating additional energy.

- Muscle Fatigue: Respiratory muscles work harder to maintain adequate airflow, leading to muscle fatigue and heightened energy consumption.

- Reduced Stamina: Individuals may experience diminished endurance and tolerance for physical activities, further limiting energy reserves.

Understanding these challenges is crucial for devising effective strategies to conserve energy and improve daily functioning.

Strategies for Conserving Energy

1. Pacing Activities

Pacing involves breaking tasks into smaller, manageable segments and alternating periods of activity with rest. This approach prevents overexertion, conserves energy, and mitigates the risk of symptom exacerbation:

- Task Segmentation: Divide larger tasks into smaller steps and intersperse breaks between activities to prevent fatigue.

- Task Prioritization: Focus on essential activities and spread them throughout the day to avoid excessive strain during peak energy periods.

2. Optimizing Daily Routine

Efficiently organizing daily activities helps minimize energy expenditure and maximize productivity:

- Scheduled Rest Periods: Plan regular breaks to recharge and prevent exhaustion. Use relaxation techniques such as deep breathing or meditation during breaks to alleviate stress and conserve energy.

- Use of Mobility Aids: Consider utilizing assistive devices like wheeled carts or walkers to transport heavy items or reduce physical exertion during tasks.

3. Conserving Physical Energy

Implementing practical tips to diminish physical strain supports energy conservation:

- Simplifying Tasks: Streamline daily routines by arranging frequently used items within easy reach. Utilize tools with ergonomic designs to minimize strain on joints and muscles.

- Environmental Adjustments: Arrange furniture and household items for optimal accessibility and comfort. Utilize chairs with supportive backs and cushions to alleviate discomfort during prolonged sitting.

4. Managing Breathlessness

Strategies to manage breathlessness aid in conserving energy and enhancing overall well-being:

- Breathing Techniques: Practice techniques such as diaphragmatic breathing and pursed lip breathing to enhance oxygen efficiency and reduce respiratory effort.

- Optimal Positioning: Maintain a comfortable posture and use pillows or cushions to support the head and chest, facilitating easier breathing and conserving energy.

5. Utilizing Technology and Tools

Incorporating assistive technologies and adaptive aids helps conserve energy and foster independence:

- Home Modifications: Install grab bars in bathrooms, ramps for wheelchair accessibility, and automated devices for controlling lights and appliances to minimize physical exertion.

- Use of Assistive Devices: Explore options like reachers, jar openers, and dressing aids to simplify daily tasks and conserve energy.

6. Strategic Planning and Prioritization

Effective time management and prioritization play pivotal roles in conserving mental and emotional energy:

- Establishing Daily Plans: Develop a structured daily schedule that balances activities with ample rest periods. Prioritize tasks based on importance and allocate energy accordingly.

- Delegation of Responsibilities: Delegate tasks to family members, caregivers, or support networks to lighten the workload and conserve personal energy reserves.

7. Embracing Adaptive Strategies

Adapting to fluctuating energy levels and adjusting expectations facilitates effective energy conservation:

- Flexibility: Modify daily routines and activities based on current energy levels and symptoms. Embrace adaptations as necessary to maintain comfort and prevent exhaustion.

- Self-Care Practices: Emphasize self-care activities such as maintaining hydration, balanced nutrition, and adequate sleep to bolster overall energy levels and well-being.

Integrating Energy Conservation with The COPD Solution Program

The COPD Solution Program underscores the integration of energy-saving techniques to optimize disease management and enhance quality of life:

- Personalized Approach: Customize energy conservation strategies to align with individual needs and preferences, taking into account specific COPD symptoms and lifestyle factors.

- Collaboration with Healthcare Providers: Forge a close partnership with healthcare providers to devise a tailored plan for conserving energy, managing symptoms, and improving overall well-being.

- Education and Support: Receive comprehensive guidance on implementing energy-saving techniques, including practical tips, educational resources, and access to support networks for coping with challenges associated with COPD.

Conclusion

Embracing and implementing energy conservation strategies are pivotal in effectively managing COPD and elevating quality of life. By embracing techniques such as pacing activities, optimizing daily routines, conserving physical energy, managing breathlessness, utilizing assistive technologies, strategic planning, and adapting to evolving needs, individuals can mitigate fatigue, reduce symptom exacerbation, and enhance overall well-being. The integration of energy conservation principles with The COPD Solution Program provides a comprehensive framework for achieving these objectives, empowering individuals to take charge of their condition and lead fulfilling lives despite the obstacles posed by COPD. Through proactive management and unwavering support, individuals with COPD can optimize energy utilization, preserve independence, and experience heightened comfort and well-being on a daily basis.

CHAPTER 5: PREVENTING FLARE-UPS: OPTIMIZING MEDICATION USE

Preventing exacerbations, or flare-ups, of Chronic Obstructive Pulmonary Disease (COPD) is crucial for maintaining stability in health and quality of life. This chapter explores the importance of effectively utilizing medications to manage COPD, strategies for preventing flare-ups, and practical advice on integrating medication management into daily life. By comprehending the role of medications and adhering to The COPD Solution Program, individuals can effectively reduce the frequency and severity of exacerbations, leading to better disease control and improved well-being.

Understanding COPD Medications

Managing COPD typically involves medications aimed at relieving symptoms, improving lung function, reducing inflammation, and preventing exacerbations. The COPD Solution Program advocates for a comprehensive approach to medication management tailored to individual needs and disease severity.

Types of COPD Medications

1. Bronchodilators:

   - Short-Acting Bronchodilators: These provide rapid relief by relaxing airway muscles, improving airflow. Examples include albuterol (ProAir HFA, Ventolin HFA) and ipratropium (Atrovent).

   - Long-Acting Bronchodilators: These offer sustained relief over a longer duration, typically administered once or twice daily. Examples include long-acting beta agonists (LABAs) such as salmeterol (Serevent Diskus) and formoterol (Foradil, Perforomist), and long-acting anticholinergics (LAMAs) like tiotropium (Spiriva) and aclidinium (Tudorza Pressair).

2. Anti-Inflammatory Medications:

- Inhaled Corticosteroids (ICS): These medications reduce airway inflammation and are often used in combination with bronchodilators for moderate to severe COPD. Examples include fluticasone (Flovent HFA) and budesonide (Pulmicort Flexhaler).

- Combination Therapy: Some medications combine bronchodilators and corticosteroids to provide enhanced symptom relief and reduce exacerbation risk. Examples include fluticasone/salmeterol (Advair Diskus) and budesonide/formoterol (Symbicort).

3. Other Medications:

- Phosphodiesterase-4 Inhibitors: Medications like roflumilast (Daliresp) reduce inflammation and relax airways, typically prescribed for severe COPD with chronic bronchitis.

- Antibiotics: Prescribed during exacerbations to treat bacterial infections that can worsen COPD symptoms.

Importance of Medication Adherence

Adhering to prescribed medications is critical for effectively managing COPD and preventing exacerbations. The COPD Solution Program highlights several benefits of medication adherence:

- Symptom Control: Regular medication use helps maintain stable lung function and reduces the frequency of symptoms such as coughing, wheezing, and shortness of breath.

- Exacerbation Prevention: Proper adherence lowers the risk of exacerbations, reducing emergency visits or hospitalizations.

- Improved Quality of Life: By controlling symptoms and minimizing exacerbation risk, adherence enhances overall well-being and enables greater engagement in daily activities.

Strategies for Optimizing Medication Use

1. Understanding Medication Regimens

Become familiar with prescribed medications, including their purpose, dosage, and administration instructions:

- Follow Prescribed Schedule: Take medications as directed by your healthcare provider, whether daily, twice daily, or as needed for rescue medications.
- Proper Inhaler Technique: Learn correct inhaler techniques for optimal medication delivery. Techniques vary among metered-dose inhalers (MDIs),

dry powder inhalers (DPIs), and nebulizers.

- Storage and Handling: Store medications according to instructions (e.g., room temperature, protected from light and moisture). Ensure inhalers and nebulizers are maintained correctly to retain effectiveness.

2. Developing a Medication Management Plan

Create a personalized medication management plan in collaboration with your healthcare provider:

- Medication Schedule: Establish a routine for taking medications to ensure consistency and adherence.
- Monitoring and Feedback: Regularly assess medication effectiveness and

discuss any concerns or side effects with your healthcare provider.
- Emergency Plan: Develop an action plan for managing exacerbations, including steps to take and when to seek medical assistance.

3. Benefits of Combination Therapy

For individuals with moderate to severe COPD, combination therapy (e.g., LABA/ICS or LAMA/LABA) offers enhanced symptom control and prevention of exacerbations:

- Synergistic Effects: Combining medications with different mechanisms (bronchodilation and anti-inflammatory) provides comprehensive symptom relief.

- Single-Inhaler Options: Simplify medication regimens and improve adherence with single-inhaler combination therapies.

4. Monitoring and Adjusting Medications

Regularly evaluate medication effectiveness and adjust treatment plans as needed:

- Symptom Monitoring: Keep track of COPD symptoms and exacerbation frequency to assess medication efficacy.
- Lung Function Tests: Periodic spirometry tests help gauge lung function and adjust medication dosages accordingly.

- Healthcare Provider Collaboration: Schedule regular follow-up appointments to review treatment progress, discuss changes in symptoms, and adjust medications when necessary.

5. Lifestyle Integration

Incorporate medication adherence into daily routines alongside healthy lifestyle habits:

- Smoking Cessation: Quit smoking to optimize medication effectiveness and slow disease progression.
- Physical Activity: Engage in regular exercise as recommended to improve lung function and overall health.
- Nutrition: Maintain a balanced diet to support respiratory health and overall well-being.

Integrating Medication Management with The COPD Solution Program

The COPD Solution Program integrates medication management as a cornerstone of disease management and prevention:

- Personalized Treatment Plans: Customize medication regimens based on individual needs, considering COPD severity, symptoms, and lifestyle factors.
- Education and Support: Receive comprehensive education on COPD medications, including benefits, side effects, and proper usage techniques.

- Collaboration with Healthcare Providers: Work closely with healthcare providers to monitor medication effectiveness, adjust treatment plans, and address any concerns or questions.

Conclusion

Effectively managing COPD and preventing exacerbations relies on using medications appropriately and adhering to prescribed treatment regimens. By understanding the role of medications in controlling symptoms, improving lung function, and minimizing exacerbation risk, individuals can achieve better disease control and enhance their quality of life. The COPD Solution Program provides a structured approach to medication management, emphasizing personalized treatment plans, proper inhaler techniques, regular monitoring, and integration with lifestyle habits. Through proactive medication management and collaboration with healthcare providers, individuals with COPD can optimize treatment outcomes, reduce exacerbation frequency, and maintain greater stability in health and well-being. By committing to medication adherence and incorporating these strategies into daily life, individuals can effectively manage their condition and achieve a higher level of comfort and independence despite the challenges posed by COPD.

CHAPTER 6: ATTENDING PULMONARY REHABILITATION: STRENGTHENING YOUR RESPIRATORY HEALTH

Participating in pulmonary rehabilitation (PR) represents a pivotal step in the holistic management of Chronic Obstructive Pulmonary Disease (COPD). This chapter delves into the significance of PR, its advantages, what participants can anticipate from PR programs, and practical guidance on seamlessly integrating PR into daily routines. By embracing PR in conjunction with The COPD Solution Program, individuals can bolster their respiratory function, augment their exercise endurance, and achieve an enhanced overall quality of life.

Understanding Pulmonary Rehabilitation

Pulmonary rehabilitation is a structured program designed to ameliorate the physical and emotional well-being of individuals grappling with chronic respiratory conditions such as COPD. It employs a multidisciplinary approach encompassing exercise training, education on COPD management, breathing techniques, and psychological support. The COPD Solution Program integrates PR as a fundamental element of disease management to aid individuals in optimizing their respiratory health and coping adeptly with the challenges associated with COPD.

Benefits of Pulmonary Rehabilitation

1. Enhanced Exercise Capacity: PR programs concentrate on augmenting physical stamina and exercise tolerance

through tailored exercise regimens. Participants progressively bolster their capability to engage in daily activities with diminished exertion and fatigue.

2. Improved Management of Breathlessness: Participants acquire proficiency in effective breathing techniques like pursed lip breathing and diaphragmatic breathing, which alleviate breathlessness during physical exertion and enhance overall oxygen utilization efficiency.

3. Education on COPD Management: PR imparts vital knowledge about COPD, encompassing its symptoms, medications, and strategies for mitigating flare-ups. This equips individuals with the understanding

needed to effectively monitor and control their condition.

4. Psychosocial Support: PR programs furnish emotional sustenance and coping mechanisms to address the psychological impact of COPD. This encompasses stress management techniques, counseling sessions, and communal support among participants, fostering a sense of camaraderie.

5. Enhanced Quality of Life: By bolstering physical fitness, alleviating symptoms, and providing psychological bolstering, PR significantly enhances overall quality of life for individuals grappling with COPD.

What to Expect from Pulmonary Rehabilitation Programs

Structure of PR Programs

PR programs typically span several weeks and encompass:

- Initial Evaluation: A thorough assessment conducted by healthcare professionals to gauge baseline fitness, lung function, and individual requirements.

- Exercise Training: Supervised sessions incorporating aerobic exercises (such as walking or cycling) and strength training to bolster respiratory muscle vigor and endurance.

- Educational Sessions: Classes addressing topics like COPD management, medication regimens, nutritional guidance, and coping strategies.

- Breathing Techniques: Instruction on adopting effective breathing techniques to optimize oxygenation and mitigate breathlessness.

- Psychosocial Support: Counseling sessions, support groups, and techniques for stress management tailored to address the emotional facets of coping with COPD.

Personalized Care

PR programs are tailored to suit individual needs, taking into account factors like the severity of COPD, overall health status, and personal aspirations:

- Customized Exercise Plans: Exercises are customized to align with the participant's fitness levels and progression objectives, ensuring safety and efficacy.

- Accessible Education: Information is imparted in a clear, understandable manner to empower participants in the self-management of their condition.

- Ongoing Monitoring: Regular evaluations track progress and facilitate modifications to the program as warranted by individual progress.

Integrating Pulmonary Rehabilitation with The COPD Solution Program

Tailored Treatment Plans

The COPD Solution Program integrates PR as an integral component of individualized treatment plans:

- Collaboration with Healthcare Providers: Close collaboration with healthcare providers facilitates the recommendation of PR based on individual requirements and the facilitation of enrollment in suitable programs.

- Alignment of PR Objectives: Harmonizing PR goals with broader COPD management strategies enhances outcomes and bolsters overall health.

Educational and Supportive Components

- Comprehensive Instruction: Provision of comprehensive information about the benefits of PR, what to expect from participation, and how it complements overall COPD management.

- Support Networks: Encouragement of participation in support groups and provision of access to resources that foster ongoing support and education.

Integration into Daily Life

- Long-Term Advantages: Emphasis on the enduring benefits of PR in sustaining physical fitness, managing symptoms, and forestalling exacerbations.

- Sustainable Practices: Encouragement of the integration of PR principles into daily routines to sustain improvements in respiratory health and overall well-being.

Practical Advice for Integrating Pulmonary Rehabilitation

1. Commitment to Attendance
Prioritize attendance at PR sessions and adhere to the recommended schedule to maximize benefits.

2. Active Engagement in Exercises

Participate actively in exercise sessions, adhering to guidance from healthcare professionals to optimize effectiveness.

3. Consistent Practice of Breathing Techniques

Regularly practice the breathing techniques learned during PR sessions to effectively manage breathlessness and optimize oxygen intake.

4. Application of Educational Insights

Apply the knowledge gained from educational sessions to better manage COPD symptoms, adhere to medication regimens, and implement lifestyle adjustments.

5. Utilization of Supportive Resources

Engage with support groups, counseling services, and educational materials provided through PR to enhance coping skills and emotional well-being.

Conclusion

Engagement in pulmonary rehabilitation constitutes a critical component of effectively managing COPD and enhancing quality of life. By participating in structured exercise programs, acquiring essential COPD management skills, and benefiting from psychological support, individuals can fortify their respiratory health, augment their capacity for physical activity, and alleviate symptom burdens. Integration of pulmonary rehabilitation with The COPD Solution Program embodies a comprehensive approach to managing the disease, underpinned by personalized care, education, and the integration of healthy lifestyle practices. Through commitment to PR and collaboration with healthcare providers, individuals with COPD can achieve favorable outcomes, preserve their independence, and experience heightened comfort and well-being in daily life. Pulmonary rehabilitation not only promotes physical fitness but also empowers individuals to proactively manage their condition, fostering optimism and enhancing overall health despite the challenges posed by COPD.

CHAPTER 7: STOPPING SMOKING: ESSENTIAL IN COPD MANAGEMENT

Smoking cessation plays a crucial role in effectively managing Chronic Obstructive Pulmonary Disease (COPD). This chapter delves into the profound impact of smoking on COPD, the benefits of quitting, effective strategies for smoking cessation, and practical advice on integrating smoking cessation into daily life. By prioritizing smoking cessation alongside The

COPD Solution Program, individuals can significantly slow disease progression, alleviate symptoms, and enhance their overall quality of life.

Understanding the Impact of Smoking on COPD

Smoking stands as the predominant cause of COPD, contributing to approximately 85-90% of cases. Tobacco smoke contains harmful chemicals that inflict damage on the lungs and airways, leading to persistent inflammation, narrowing of the air passages, and irreversible lung impairment over time. For individuals living with COPD, continued smoking exacerbates symptoms such as persistent coughing, wheezing, and breathlessness, while also accelerating the progression of the disease.

Effects of Smoking on COPD:

1. Airway Inflammation: Tobacco smoke irritates and inflames the airways, triggering chronic inflammation that obstructs airflow and impairs lung function.

2. Lung Damage: Smoking progressively destroys the delicate lung tissues and reduces their elasticity, making it increasingly challenging to breathe over time.

3. Exacerbation Risk: Smokers with COPD face heightened risks of frequent and severe exacerbations, which often necessitate hospitalizations and further deteriorate lung function.

4. Reduced Treatment Efficacy: Continued smoking diminishes the effectiveness of medications and therapies aimed at managing COPD symptoms and improving lung function.

Understanding these adverse effects underscores the urgency and significance of quitting smoking to mitigate disease progression and achieve better health outcomes.

Benefits of Smoking Cessation

Quitting smoking at any stage of COPD offers substantial health benefits and positively impacts disease management:

1. Slowed Disease Progression: Cessation of smoking halts the decline in lung function and lowers the risk of developing complications associated with COPD.

2. Improved Lung Function: Within weeks to months of quitting, lung function begins to improve as inflammation subsides and lung tissue begins to heal.

3. Symptom Relief: Many individuals experience diminished coughing, reduced wheezing, and lessened shortness of breath, leading to enhanced comfort and improved quality of life.

4. Lower Exacerbation Risk: Non-smokers with COPD typically experience fewer and less severe exacerbations, resulting in reduced need for emergency medical care and hospitalizations.

5. Enhanced Treatment Response: Smoking cessation enhances the effectiveness of medications and therapies prescribed for COPD management.

These benefits underscore smoking cessation as a pivotal intervention in COPD management, offering tangible improvements in health and well-being.

Strategies for Smoking Cessation

Effective smoking cessation strategies encompass a blend of behavioral interventions, support systems, and pharmacological aids designed to address both the physical and psychological aspects of nicotine addiction:

1. Behavioral Interventions

- Counseling: Individual or group counseling sessions offer personalized support, guidance, and coping strategies tailored to the individual's needs.

- Behavioral Therapy: Cognitive-behavioral techniques help identify triggers, modify smoking behaviors, and develop healthier coping mechanisms.

2. Nicotine Replacement Therapy (NRT)

- Nicotine Patches: Provide a steady, controlled release of nicotine to alleviate withdrawal symptoms and reduce cravings.

- Nicotine Gum or Lozenges: Offer on-demand relief for cravings and help manage oral fixation associated with smoking.

3. Prescription Medications

- Bupropion (Zyban): Helps reduce nicotine cravings and withdrawal symptoms by affecting brain chemistry.

- Varenicline (Chantix): Reduces the pleasurable effects of nicotine and alleviates withdrawal symptoms.

4. Support Systems

- Support Groups: Engaging with peers who are also quitting smoking provides encouragement, shared experiences, and accountability.

- Family and Friends: Enlist the support of loved ones to provide encouragement, understanding, and motivation throughout the quitting process.

5. Lifestyle Changes

- Avoid Triggers: Identify and avoid situations, places, or activities that trigger the urge to smoke.

- Healthy Substitutions: Substitute smoking with healthier habits such as physical exercise, hobbies, or relaxation techniques to manage stress and cravings effectively.

6. Setting Goals and Rewards

- Goal Setting: Establish realistic, achievable goals for quitting smoking, such as reducing cigarette consumption gradually or setting a quit date.

- Reward System: Celebrate milestones and achievements with rewards that reinforce progress and motivate continued efforts towards cessation.

Integrating Smoking Cessation with The COPD Solution Program

Personalized Support

The COPD Solution Program integrates smoking cessation as a cornerstone of personalized treatment plans:

- Healthcare Provider Collaboration: Collaborate closely with healthcare providers to develop personalized cessation strategies aligned with COPD management goals.

- Education and Counseling: Provide comprehensive education on the benefits of smoking cessation, withdrawal symptoms, and effective coping strategies to empower individuals throughout their quit journey.

Lifestyle Adjustment

- Long-Term Health Focus: Emphasize the enduring health benefits of quitting smoking in managing COPD and enhancing overall quality of life.

- Sustainable Practices: Support the integration of smoking cessation strategies into daily routines to maintain cessation and prevent relapse effectively.

Practical Advice for Quitting Smoking

1. Commitment to Quitting

Make a steadfast commitment to quit smoking and set a quit date to initiate the cessation process.

2. Utilize Support Resources

Take advantage of counseling services, support groups, and pharmacological aids to enhance the likelihood of successful cessation.

3. Develop Coping Strategies

Learn and practice coping strategies to manage cravings, stress, and withdrawal symptoms effectively.

4. Adopt Healthy Lifestyle Habits

Embrace healthy habits such as regular exercise, balanced nutrition, and stress-reducing activities to support smoking cessation efforts.

5. Monitor Progress

Regularly assess progress, celebrate successes, and seek assistance if encountering challenges or setbacks during the quitting process.

Conclusion

Quitting smoking is an essential step in managing COPD effectively and improving overall quality of life. By quitting smoking, individuals can significantly mitigate disease progression, alleviate symptoms, and enhance lung function. The integration of smoking cessation with The COPD Solution Program offers a comprehensive approach to disease management, emphasizing personalized support, education, and sustainable lifestyle adjustments. Through commitment to smoking cessation strategies and collaboration with healthcare providers, individuals with COPD can achieve substantial health benefits, enhance their well-being, and enjoy a better quality of life free from the harmful effects of smoking. Quitting smoking not only improves physical health but also empowers individuals to take control of their condition, fostering optimism and resilience in managing COPD despite its challenges.

CHAPTER 8: RECIPES: EATING FOR IMPROVED RESPIRATORY HEALTH

Managing and overcoming Chronic Obstructive Pulmonary Disease (COPD) involves harnessing the power of nutrition. This chapter delves into recipes tailored to support lung function and overall well-being. By incorporating these nourishing and delightful meals into your daily routine alongside The COPD Solution Program, you can optimize lung function, alleviate symptoms, and enhance your quality of life.

Breakfast Recipes: Energizing Your Day

Whole Grain Bowl

Ingredients:
- 1/2 cup cooked quinoa
- 1/4 cup chopped almonds
- 1 tablespoon chia seeds
- 1/2 cup mixed berries (blueberries, strawberries)
- 1 tablespoon honey or maple syrup
- 1/2 cup almond milk or yogurt (optional)

Instructions:
1. Combine quinoa, almonds, chia seeds, and mixed berries in a bowl.
2. Drizzle with honey or maple syrup for sweetness.
3. Add almond milk or yogurt if desired.
4. Mix well to enjoy a nutritious blend rich in whole grains, nuts, seeds, and antioxidants.

Greek Granola On-the-Go

Ingredients:
- 1 cup rolled oats
- 1/4 cup chopped walnuts or almonds
- 1/4 cup pumpkin seeds
- 1/4 cup dried cranberries or raisins
- 1/2 teaspoon cinnamon
- 1/4 cup honey or agave syrup
- 1/4 cup plain Greek yogurt

Instructions:
1. Preheat oven to 325°F (165°C).
2. Mix oats, nuts, pumpkin seeds, dried cranberries, and cinnamon in a bowl.
3. Drizzle honey or agave syrup over the mixture and stir well.
4. Spread evenly on a parchment-lined baking sheet.
5. Bake for 20-25 minutes until golden brown, stirring halfway.
6. Cool completely and store in an airtight container.
7. Serve with Greek yogurt for a protein-packed breakfast option.

Avocado Breakfast Eggs

Ingredients:
- 2 eggs
- 1 ripe avocado

- Salt and pepper to taste
- Fresh herbs (optional, for garnish)

Instructions:
1. Halve the avocado and remove the pit.
2. Scoop out some avocado to enlarge the hole for the egg.
3. Crack an egg into each avocado half.
4. Season with salt and pepper.
5. Bake at 400°F (200°C) for 10-15 minutes until eggs are cooked.
6. Garnish with herbs and serve warm.

Lunch Recipes: Nourishing and Satisfying

Tasty Grilled Cheese

Ingredients:
- 2 slices whole grain bread
- 1/2 cup shredded cheddar cheese
- 1 tablespoon butter or olive oil

Instructions:
1. Heat a skillet over medium heat.
2. Butter one side of each bread slice.
3. Place one slice, buttered side down, on the skillet.
4. Top with cheddar and cover with the other slice, buttered side up.

5. Cook for 3-4 minutes per side until golden brown and cheese melts.
6. Cut into halves or quarters and serve hot.

Homemade Guacamole

Ingredients:
- 2 ripe avocados
- 1/2 small red onion, finely diced
- 1 tomato, seeded and diced
- 1 clove garlic, minced
- Juice of 1 lime
- Salt and pepper to taste
- Fresh cilantro (optional, for garnish)

Instructions:
1. Scoop avocado into a bowl and mash with a fork.
2. Stir in onion, tomato, garlic, lime juice, salt, and pepper.

3. Adjust seasoning as needed.

4. Garnish with cilantro and serve with whole grain chips or alongside grilled meats.

Ham and Cream Cheese Roll

Ingredients:
- 4 slices lean ham
- 4 tablespoons low-fat cream cheese
- 1/2 cucumber, cut into thin strips
- Fresh spinach leaves

Instructions:

1. Lay ham slices flat.

2. Spread cream cheese evenly on each slice.

3. Layer cucumber strips and spinach leaves on top.

4. Roll tightly and slice into bite-sized rolls.

5. Serve chilled as a protein-rich lunch option.

Dinner Recipes: Flavorful and Nutrient-Rich

Lime Chicken and Rice

Ingredients:
- 4 boneless, skinless chicken breasts
- Juice and zest of 2 limes
- 2 tablespoons olive oil
- 2 garlic cloves, minced
- 1 teaspoon ground cumin
- Salt and pepper to taste
- 2 cups cooked brown rice
- Fresh cilantro (optional, for garnish)

Instructions:
1. Whisk lime juice, zest, olive oil, garlic, cumin, salt, and pepper.
2. Marinate chicken for at least 30 minutes.
3. Grill or pan-fry chicken until cooked through.
4. Slice and serve over brown rice.
5. Garnish with cilantro.

Quinoa and Black Bean Salad

Ingredients:
- 1 cup quinoa, cooked and cooled
- 1 can (15 oz) black beans, rinsed and drained
- 1 red bell pepper, diced
- 1 cup cherry tomatoes, halved
- 1/4 cup red onion, finely chopped
- 1/4 cup cilantro, chopped
- Juice of 1 lime

- 2 tablespoons olive oil
- Salt and pepper to taste
- Avocado slices (optional, for garnish)

Instructions:
1. Combine quinoa, beans, bell pepper, tomatoes, onion, and cilantro.
2. Whisk lime juice, olive oil, salt, and pepper.
3. Toss salad with dressing.
4. Chill before serving.
5. Garnish with avocado.

Brown Sugar Glazed Salmon

Ingredients:
- 4 salmon fillets
- 1/4 cup brown sugar
- 2 tablespoons soy sauce
- 1 tablespoon Dijon mustard
- 1 tablespoon olive oil

- 2 garlic cloves, minced
- Salt and pepper to taste
- Lemon wedges (optional, for serving)

Instructions:
1. Preheat oven to 400°F (200°C).
2. Whisk brown sugar, soy sauce, mustard, olive oil, garlic, salt, and pepper.
3. Brush salmon with glaze.
4. Bake until flaky.
5. Serve with lemon.

Desserts/Smoothies: Refreshing and Nutrient-Packed

Orange Dream Smoothie

Ingredients:
- 1 cup orange juice
- 1/2 cup Greek yogurt
- 1 frozen banana
- 1/2 cup frozen mango chunks
- 1 tablespoon honey or maple syrup (optional)

Instructions:
1. Blend orange juice, yogurt, banana, and mango.
2. Add honey or syrup for sweetness.
3. Serve cold.

Popeye's Favorite Spinach Smoothie

Ingredients:
- 1 cup spinach leaves
- 1/2 cup frozen pineapple chunks
- 1/2 cup frozen mango chunks
- 1/2 banana
- 1 cup coconut water or almond milk

Instructions:
1. Blend spinach, pineapple, mango, banana, and liquid.
2. Adjust thickness.
3. Serve chilled.

Protein Fruit Smoothie

Ingredients:
- 1 cup mixed berries
- 1/2 cup Greek yogurt
- 1/2 cup almond or soy milk

- 1 scoop protein powder (optional)
- 1 tablespoon chia seeds (optional)
- Honey or syrup (optional)

Instructions:

1. Blend berries, yogurt, milk, powder, and seeds.
2. Adjust thickness.
3. Serve cold.

Cucumber and Honeydew Smoothie

Ingredients:
- 1 cup cucumber, diced
- 1 cup honeydew melon, diced
- 1/2 cup Greek yogurt
- Juice of 1 lime
- 1 tablespoon honey
- Ice cubes (optional)

Instructions:
1. Blend cucumber, melon, yogurt, lime, and honey.
2. Add ice for chill.
3. Serve cold.

Smoothie on the Beach

Ingredients:
- 1 cup pineapple, fresh or frozen
- 1/2 cup mango, fresh or frozen
- 1/2 cup coconut water
- Juice of 1 lime
- 1 tablespoon shredded coconut (optional)

Instructions:
1. Blend pineapple, mango, water, and lime.
2. Garnish with coconut.
3. Serve chilled.

Conclusion

By integrating these recipes into your daily regimen through The COPD Solution Program, you can significantly enhance respiratory health. These meals provide essential nutrients, bolster immunity, and sustain energy. Focus on whole grains, lean proteins, healthy fats, and antioxidant-rich fruits and vegetables to manage COPD symptoms and optimize lung function.

Consistency is key. Select recipes aligned with your taste preferences and dietary requirements. Experiment with ingredients to maintain meal variety and enjoyment. Alongside medication, exercise, and medical oversight, these nutritious recipes contribute to a holistic approach to COPD management.

Prioritize your health with informed food choices. Embrace these recipes, relish their flavors, and embrace the benefits they offer in your journey to improved respiratory health. Here's to nourishing yourself well, breathing easier, and living fully with COPD.

CHAPTER 9: PRACTICING YOGA FOR MANAGING COPD

In the pursuit of managing and overcoming Chronic Obstructive Pulmonary Disease (COPD), incorporating holistic practices such as yoga can significantly enhance overall well-being. Part 2 of our ebook, "The COPD Solution Program," explores complementary approaches that synergize with medical treatments to improve respiratory function and quality of life. Among these approaches, yoga stands out for its gentle yet powerful impact on breathing, physical flexibility, and mental health.

Understanding Yoga and COPD

Originating from ancient India, yoga integrates physical postures (asanas), breathing techniques (pranayama), and meditation to foster physical and mental balance. For individuals living with COPD, yoga offers structured methods to enhance lung capacity, reduce stress, and cultivate inner calm amidst respiratory challenges.

Benefits of Yoga for COPD Patients

1. Improved Respiratory Function: Yoga encourages mindful breathing exercises that enhance lung capacity and efficiency. Techniques like diaphragmatic breathing help COPD patients utilize their lungs more effectively, reducing the effort required for each breath.

2. Enhanced Physical Flexibility: COPD often leads to chest stiffness and reduced physical activity. Yoga postures gently stretch and strengthen muscles, improving flexibility and easing muscle tension associated with breathing difficulties.

3. Stress Reduction: COPD can cause significant anxiety and stress, exacerbating symptoms. Yoga promotes relaxation through deep breathing and meditation, lowering cortisol levels and fostering a calmer state of mind.

4. Improved Quality of Life: Regular yoga practice has been shown to enhance overall well-being in COPD patients. It improves mood, sleep quality, and energy levels, offering a holistic approach to managing the disease.

Yoga Practices for COPD Patients

1. Pranayama (Breathing Techniques)

Pranayama forms the core of yoga practice for COPD management, focusing on controlled breathing patterns that alleviate respiratory distress and enhance oxygenation. Effective techniques include:

- Diaphragmatic Breathing (Belly Breathing): Sit or lie down comfortably, placing one hand on your abdomen and the other on your chest. Inhale deeply through your nose, allowing your abdomen to rise as your lungs fill with air. Exhale slowly through pursed lips, feeling your abdomen fall. Repeat, focusing on the smooth flow of air and relaxation of chest muscles.

- Alternate Nostril Breathing (Nadi Shodhana): Sit comfortably with a straight spine. Close your right nostril with your thumb and inhale deeply through your left nostril. Close the left nostril with your ring finger, release the thumb, and exhale through the right nostril. Inhale through the right nostril, close it with your thumb, release the left nostril, and exhale through the left. Repeat this cycle, maintaining a steady, controlled breath.

2. Yoga Asanas (Postures)

Yoga postures are adapted to suit the needs of COPD patients, focusing on gentle movements that enhance lung function and flexibility without strain. Some beneficial asanas include:

- Sukhasana (Easy Pose): Sit cross-legged with a straight spine, hands resting on knees or in lap. Close your eyes and focus on deep, even breaths to relax the mind and improve posture.

- Tadasana (Mountain Pose): Stand tall with feet hip-width apart. Inhale deeply as you raise arms overhead, palms facing each other. Stretch upwards while maintaining a steady breath to improve lung capacity and posture.

- Setu Bandhasana (Bridge Pose): Lie on your back with knees bent and feet hip-width apart. Inhale, lift hips towards the ceiling, keeping shoulders and feet grounded. Hold briefly, then exhale slowly while lowering back down. This pose strengthens chest muscles and improves lung expansion.

3. Meditation and Relaxation

COPD often brings emotional challenges like anxiety and depression. Meditation and relaxation techniques practiced in yoga promote mental clarity and emotional resilience. Even a few minutes of daily meditation can significantly reduce stress levels and improve overall well-being.

Integrating Yoga into Your COPD Management Plan

To integrate yoga effectively into your COPD management plan, follow these guidelines:

1. Consult Your Healthcare Provider: Before starting any new exercise regimen, especially yoga, consult your healthcare provider, particularly if you have severe COPD or other health conditions.

2. Start Slowly and Gradually: Begin with gentle yoga poses and breathing exercises. Listen to your body and avoid overexertion.

3. Practice Consistently: Aim for regular practice, even if only for a few minutes each day. Consistency is key to experiencing the benefits of yoga.

4. Adapt Poses as Needed: Modify poses to suit your comfort and ability. Use props like cushions or blocks for support as necessary.

5. Stay Mindful: During practice, focus on the present moment. Be aware of your breath, body sensations, and thoughts without judgment.

Conclusion

Incorporating yoga into your COPD management plan through Part 2 of "The COPD Solution Program" offers a holistic approach to improving respiratory function, reducing stress, and enhancing overall quality of life. By regularly practicing pranayama, gentle asanas, and meditation, you can cultivate resilience on your journey to managing and overcoming COPD. Remember, each breath counts towards better health, and yoga serves as a supportive companion along this path.

In the upcoming chapter, we will explore nutritional strategies that complement yoga and medical treatments, further optimizing your COPD management plan. Stay tuned for insights into dietary choices that support respiratory health and overall well-being.

CHAPTER 10: STAYING CONNECTED IN YOUR COPD JOURNEY

In the fight against Chronic Obstructive Pulmonary Disease (COPD), maintaining connections and support systems is pivotal for improving quality of life and effectively managing the complexities associated with the condition. Part 2 of our ebook, "The COPD Solution Program," underscores the critical role of staying connected—both socially and emotionally—to fortify resilience and nurture a positive mindset throughout your COPD journey.

Understanding the Importance of Staying Connected

Living with COPD often leads to feelings of isolation and loneliness, especially as symptoms progress and daily activities become more challenging. Staying connected goes beyond mere social interaction; it encompasses emotional support, access to information, and resources that significantly influence your ability to cope and thrive.

Benefits of Staying Connected for COPD Patients

1. Emotional Support: Establishing and maintaining connections with family, friends, support groups, and healthcare providers provides essential emotional support. Sharing experiences and emotions with individuals who understand can alleviate feelings of isolation and enhance mental well-being.

2. Access to Information: Being connected ensures you stay informed about the latest advancements in COPD treatments, management strategies, and lifestyle adjustments. This knowledge

empowers patients to make informed decisions about their health and treatment plans.

3. Encouragement and Motivation: Connections with others offer encouragement and motivation, particularly during difficult times. Supportive relationships inspire COPD patients to adhere to treatment regimens, engage in physical activities, and adopt healthier lifestyle habits.

4. Reduced Stress and Anxiety: Social connections and support networks help alleviate the stress and anxiety associated with COPD. Having someone to confide in and lean on during challenging moments provides comfort and reassurance.

Strategies for Maintaining Connections

1. Family and Friends

Family and friends serve as the primary support network for COPD patients. Strengthen these connections with the following approaches:

- Open Communication: Engage in open discussions with loved ones about your COPD, including symptoms, treatment plans, and how they can offer support.

- Quality Time: Spend meaningful time together engaging in activities that you enjoy and can manage comfortably with your condition.

- Education: Educate your family and friends about COPD by sharing reliable information and resources. This helps them better understand your needs and provide effective support.

2. Support Groups and Communities

Participating in COPD support groups and communities offers invaluable peer support and shared experiences. Benefit from these connections in the following ways:

- Peer Support: Interact with others who share similar experiences. Exchange tips, coping strategies, and words of encouragement.

- Online Engagement: Join online forums and social media groups dedicated to COPD. These platforms provide a convenient way to connect with individuals globally facing similar challenges.

- Local Support Networks: Seek out COPD support groups within your community or through healthcare organizations. Attend meetings or events to build connections and access local resources.

3. Healthcare Providers and Specialists

Maintain regular contact with your healthcare team to optimize your COPD management and treatment:

- Scheduled Check-ups: Attend all scheduled appointments with your healthcare provider to monitor your COPD, discuss any concerns, and adjust your treatment plan as necessary.

- Ask Questions: Take an active role in your healthcare by asking questions about your condition, treatment options, and lifestyle adjustments. Understanding empowers you to participate effectively in your care.

- Adherence to Treatment: Follow your prescribed medications, therapies, and lifestyle recommendations diligently. Compliance enhances treatment efficacy and minimizes potential complications.

4. Utilizing Technology and Resources

Leverage technology and available resources to stay informed and connected:

- Telemedicine: Utilize telemedicine for convenient access to healthcare providers, particularly for routine check-ups or consultations.

- Health Apps: Use apps designed for tracking symptoms, medications, and vital signs. Some apps also offer educational resources and tools for managing COPD.

- Online Educational Platforms: Explore reputable websites and organizations dedicated to COPD. These platforms provide up-to-date information, symptom management tips, and community support.

Overcoming Challenges to Maintain Connections

While staying connected offers numerous benefits, COPD patients may face certain challenges. Here are common obstacles and strategies to overcome them:

1. Physical Limitations: Symptoms like shortness of breath and fatigue can restrict social interactions. Manage your energy levels, plan activities during periods of higher stamina, and utilize assistive devices when necessary.

2. Emotional Impact: Coping with emotional aspects such as anxiety and depression may hinder social engagement. Seek support from a therapist or counselor as needed, and stay connected with individuals who provide empathy and understanding.

3. Geographical Barriers: Living far from family or support networks can pose challenges. Maintain connections through regular phone calls, video chats, and social media to sustain meaningful relationships across distances.

4. Financial Constraints: Healthcare costs may limit access to social activities or support groups. Seek out low-cost or free community resources,

and explore online alternatives that require minimal financial commitment.

Conclusion

Staying connected in your COPD journey, as outlined in Part 2 of "The COPD Solution Program," is crucial for enhancing emotional well-being, accessing valuable information, and receiving ongoing support from family, friends, healthcare providers, and community resources. By nurturing these connections, COPD patients can navigate challenges more effectively, improve quality of life, and maintain a positive outlook on managing and overcoming the condition.

In the upcoming chapter, we will explore advanced treatment options and emerging therapies that show promise for enhancing COPD management. Stay informed about innovative developments that may further empower you on your journey toward defeating COPD.

Common Questions asked by COPD patients and Answers

What is COPD?

Answer: COPD stands for Chronic Obstructive Pulmonary Disease. It's a progressive lung disease that makes it hard to breathe due to airflow limitation. COPD includes chronic bronchitis and emphysema, often caused by smoking or exposure to lung irritants.

What are the symptoms of COPD?

Answer: Common symptoms include shortness of breath, chronic cough, wheezing, chest tightness, and excess mucus production (phlegm).

How is COPD diagnosed?

Answer: Diagnosis involves a combination of medical history, physical exam, lung function tests (spirometry), imaging studies (like chest X-rays or CT scans), and sometimes blood tests.

What causes COPD?

Answer: Smoking is the leading cause. Other causes include long-term exposure to air pollutants, occupational dusts and chemicals, genetic factors (alpha-1 antitrypsin deficiency), and respiratory infections.

Can non-smokers get COPD?

Answer: Yes, though smoking is the primary risk factor, non-smokers can develop COPD due to exposure to secondhand smoke, air pollution, occupational hazards, or genetic predisposition.

How does smoking contribute to COPD?

Answer: Smoking damages the airways and air sacs (alveoli) in the lungs, causing inflammation and narrowing of the air passages, which leads to airflow limitation and COPD.

What are the stages of COPD?

Answer: COPD is categorized into stages based on the severity of airflow limitation (measured by spirometry) and symptoms. Stages range from mild (Stage 1) to very severe (Stage 4).

Is there a cure for COPD?

Answer: Currently, there is no cure for COPD. However, treatments and lifestyle changes can help manage symptoms, slow disease progression, and improve quality of life.

How can I manage COPD symptoms at home?

Answer: Effective home management includes quitting smoking, staying active with regular exercise (under medical supervision), following a healthy diet, managing stress, and keeping up with prescribed medications.

What medications are used to treat COPD?

Answer: Medications include bronchodilators (short-acting and long-acting) to relax the muscles around the airways and corticosteroids to reduce inflammation during exacerbations.

Can I exercise if I have COPD?

Answer: Yes, regular exercise is beneficial for COPD patients. It improves lung function, strengthens muscles, and enhances overall endurance. Consult your healthcare provider for an appropriate exercise plan.

What are exacerbations of COPD?

Answer: Exacerbations are sudden flare-ups of COPD symptoms, often triggered by infections or environmental factors, leading to increased coughing, wheezing, shortness of breath, and mucus production.

How can I prevent COPD exacerbations?

Answer: To prevent exacerbations, avoid triggers (like smoking or air pollutants), get vaccinated against flu and pneumonia, adhere to your treatment plan, and promptly report any symptom changes to your healthcare provider.

What lifestyle changes can help manage COPD?

Answer: Lifestyle changes include quitting smoking, avoiding secondhand smoke and air pollutants, maintaining a healthy weight, eating a balanced diet rich in fruits and vegetables, and staying physically active.

What is oxygen therapy, and who needs it?

Answer: Oxygen therapy involves providing supplemental oxygen to maintain adequate blood oxygen levels. It's prescribed for COPD patients with low oxygen saturation levels, particularly during exertion or at rest.

How do I use inhalers properly?

Answer: Inhalers (like metered-dose inhalers and dry powder inhalers) deliver medications directly into the lungs. Proper technique involves shaking the inhaler, exhaling fully, inhaling deeply while activating the inhaler, and holding your breath for several seconds.

Are there alternative therapies for COPD?

Answer: Alternative therapies like pulmonary rehabilitation, acupuncture, and certain herbal supplements may complement conventional treatments. Discuss with your healthcare provider before starting any alternative therapies.

Can weather changes affect COPD?

Answer: Yes, extreme temperatures, humidity, and air pressure changes can worsen COPD symptoms. Dress warmly in cold weather, stay hydrated in hot weather, and avoid outdoor activities during poor air quality days.

Is there a specific diet for COPD patients?

Answer: A balanced diet with adequate protein, healthy fats, and a variety of fruits and vegetables is beneficial. Avoid excessive salt and processed foods. Some patients find smaller, more frequent meals easier to digest.

How often should I see my doctor for COPD?

Answer: Regular check-ups are crucial. Frequency depends on disease severity and stability, typically ranging from every few months to annually. Discuss a personalized schedule with your healthcare provider.

Can COPD affect mental health?

Answer: Yes, COPD can lead to anxiety, depression, and social isolation due to breathlessness and lifestyle changes. Seeking support from loved ones and healthcare providers is important.

How can I manage anxiety related to COPD?

Answer: Techniques such as relaxation exercises, meditation, deep breathing, and counseling can help manage anxiety. Discuss with your healthcare provider if anxiety significantly impacts your daily life.

Can I travel if I have COPD?

Answer: Yes, with proper planning. Pack necessary medications, oxygen if prescribed, and medical documents. Research healthcare facilities at your destination and inform your airline about any special needs.

What should I do during a COPD exacerbation?

Answer: Follow your COPD action plan provided by your healthcare provider. Increase medication use as instructed, rest, stay hydrated, monitor symptoms closely, and seek medical help if symptoms worsen.

Are there support groups for COPD patients?

Answer: Yes, joining COPD support groups provides emotional support, education, and shared experiences. Look for local groups through healthcare providers, online forums, or organizations like the American Lung Association.

Can smoking marijuana help COPD symptoms?

Answer: Smoking marijuana can worsen COPD symptoms due to respiratory irritants. Discuss alternative options for symptom relief with your healthcare provider.

What vaccines should I get if I have COPD?

Answer: Annual flu vaccines and pneumonia vaccines (such as Pneumovax and Prevnar) are recommended to prevent infections that can exacerbate COPD.

How can I improve my sleep with COPD?

Answer: Use pillows to elevate your head, maintain a regular sleep schedule, avoid large meals and caffeine before bedtime, and use prescribed medications as directed to manage symptoms that disrupt sleep.

Can I still work with COPD?

Answer: Many COPD patients continue to work with accommodations. Discuss flexible work arrangements, such as reduced hours or tasks, with your employer. Occupational therapy can help manage work-related challenges.

Can air purifiers help with COPD?

Answer: Air purifiers can reduce indoor air pollutants like dust, pet dander, and allergens, which may benefit COPD patients. Choose a purifier with a HEPA filter and regularly maintain it according to manufacturer instructions.

Should I exercise during a COPD exacerbation?

Answer: No, rest and follow your COPD action plan. Once symptoms improve, gradually resume exercise as advised by your healthcare provider to regain strength and endurance.

Can COPD cause heart problems?

Answer: COPD increases the risk of developing heart problems like heart disease and pulmonary hypertension due to strain on the heart from reduced oxygen levels and chronic inflammation.

What is pulmonary rehabilitation?

Answer: Pulmonary rehabilitation is a structured program that includes exercise training, education, and support for COPD patients to improve physical endurance, manage symptoms, and enhance quality of life.

What should I do if I run out of medication?

Answer: Contact your pharmacy or healthcare provider immediately for a refill. Running out of medication can lead to worsening symptoms or exacerbations.

Can I use a nebulizer instead of an inhaler?

Answer: Nebulizers deliver medication in mist form, which may be easier for some COPD patients to use, especially during exacerbations or for those who have difficulty coordinating inhaler use.

How can I cope with shortness of breath?

Answer: Practice pursed-lip breathing, use relaxation techniques, sit upright or lean forward, and pace activities to manage shortness of breath. Medications prescribed by your healthcare provider can also help.

What are the signs of a COPD exacerbation?

Answer: Signs include increased shortness of breath, change in sputum color or amount, increased coughing, fever, and fatigue. Promptly follow your COPD action plan if you notice these symptoms.

Can I do breathing exercises to help COPD?

Answer: Yes, breathing exercises like diaphragmatic breathing and pursed-lip breathing can improve lung function, reduce breathlessness, and enhance relaxation. Learn these techniques from a respiratory therapist or during pulmonary rehabilitation.

Can secondhand smoke worsen COPD?

Answer: Yes, exposure to secondhand smoke can irritate the airways and worsen COPD symptoms. Avoid places where smoking is allowed and ask others not to smoke indoors or near you.

Can I drink alcohol if I have COPD?

Answer: Moderate alcohol consumption may be acceptable for some COPD patients, but excessive alcohol can interact with medications, worsen symptoms, and impact overall health. Consult your healthcare provider for personalized advice.

How can I quit smoking if I have COPD?

Answer: Quitting smoking is crucial for COPD management. Ask your healthcare provider about smoking cessation programs, medications, counseling, and support groups that can increase your chances of success.

Can allergies affect COPD?

Answer: Allergies can exacerbate COPD symptoms in some patients by triggering inflammation in the airways. Avoid allergens that worsen your symptoms and discuss allergy management with your healthcare provider.

How can I manage fatigue with COPD?

Answer: Pace yourself throughout the day, prioritize activities, rest when needed, and maintain good nutrition and hydration. Address underlying causes of fatigue, such as anemia or sleep disturbances, with your healthcare provider.

Can I use oxygen therapy at home?

Answer: Yes, if prescribed by your healthcare provider. Home oxygen therapy helps maintain adequate oxygen levels in the blood and can improve quality of life for some COPD patients.

Can COPD be genetic?

Answer: In some cases, COPD can have a genetic component, such as alpha-1 antitrypsin deficiency. Genetic testing may be recommended for individuals with a family history of COPD or early-onset disease.

How can I stay active with COPD?

Answer: Engage in activities that you enjoy and can safely perform with COPD, such as walking, swimming, or tai chi. Work with a healthcare provider to develop an exercise plan tailored to your abilities and goals.

Can stress worsen COPD symptoms?

Answer: Yes, stress can trigger or exacerbate COPD symptoms. Practice stress management techniques like deep breathing, meditation, yoga, or talking with a counselor to reduce stress levels.

How can I improve my lung function with COPD?

Answer: In addition to medications, pulmonary rehabilitation, and avoiding respiratory irritants, maintaining a healthy lifestyle with regular exercise and a balanced diet can support lung function over time.

Can I still drive if I have COPD?

Answer: In most cases, COPD does not restrict driving ability. However, if symptoms significantly impair your ability to drive safely (such as severe breathlessness or dizziness), discuss with your healthcare provider and follow local regulations.

What should I do if my symptoms worsen suddenly?

Answer: Follow your COPD action plan. Increase medication use as instructed, rest, monitor your symptoms closely, and seek medical help promptly if symptoms do not improve or if you experience severe symptoms like chest pain or confusion.

These questions and answers provide comprehensive information for COPD patients to better understand their condition, manage symptoms, and improve overall quality of life. Always consult with your healthcare provider for personalized advice and treatment recommendations.

Vote of Thanks

On behalf of the entire team behind "Defeating COPD: A Comprehensive Guide to Managing and Overcoming Chronic Obstructive Pulmonary Disease," I extend my heartfelt gratitude to all those who have supported and contributed to the creation of this invaluable resource.

First and foremost, our deepest appreciation goes to the healthcare professionals, researchers, and experts in the field of COPD who have shared their knowledge and insights. Your dedication and expertise have been instrumental in shaping this comprehensive guide, providing patients and caregivers with essential information and practical strategies.

We are also immensely grateful to the patients and their families who have bravely shared their personal experiences with COPD. Your stories have added a human touch to this ebook, offering inspiration and hope to others facing similar challenges.

A special thanks goes to our publishing team and editors, whose meticulous work ensured that the content is accurate, informative, and accessible. Your commitment to excellence has made this ebook a reliable source of information for anyone affected by COPD.

Last but not least, we extend our thanks to each reader who has chosen to explore "Defeating COPD." Your interest in improving COPD management and overcoming obstacles is truly commendable. We hope this ebook serves as a valuable companion on your journey towards better health.

As we conclude, we encourage you to share your feedback and thoughts by leaving a review on Amazon. Your reviews not only help us improve but also guide others in discovering this important resource.

Thank you once again for your support, dedication, and commitment to defeating COPD. Together, we can make a difference in the lives of millions affected by this challenging condition.

Yours Sincerely,

Jessie Wiiliams

Printed in Great Britain
by Amazon